Uplift

YOUR MIND

to Lift Off

THE WEIGHT

Uplift
YOUR MIND
to Lift Off
THE WEIGHT

**A GUIDEBOOK FOR A HOLISTIC APPROACH
TO HEALTH AND WEIGHT LOSS**

Erika A. Washington

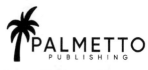

Charleston, SC
www.PalmettoPublishing.com

Uplift Your Mind to Lift Off the Weight

First Edition

Paperback ISBN: 979-8-88590-896-2

eBook ISBN: 979-8-88590-897-9

Contents

Introduction

Hello, everyone! Thank you for choosing yourself and beginning your journey to your best self! I wrote this as a guide to help you achieve and maintain your best physical self. Part of working on your physical health is also addressing the mental and emotional blocks you may have that hinder or stall your progress. Yes, weight loss and maintenance technically come down to "calories in versus calories out," *but* there is a work-around and some other things to consider. As we address these topics, I'll ask you to reflect and look within for your truth.

I've been a certified fitness instructor specializing in kickboxing for the past thirteen years. Before that, I was an exercise enthusiast who was into step aerobics, weight training, running, spin class, tai chi, belly dance, a little yoga—you name it. As a child, ballet, tap, and jazz dance were my thing. I was even on a dance team during my junior year of undergrad. I was a personal-training client for years and later had my own personal-training clients. Over the years, I have learned that it takes more than just diet and exercise to safely lose weight and keep it off. The tips I have shared in this guide have helped me lose the fifty pounds I gained during pregnancy. (I had my son at forty!) And they've helped me to keep it off without overtraining in the gym.

Some people look at me and find it hard to believe that I only do two to three forty-minute kickboxing sessions a week, yoga once a week, and belly dance once or twice a week. They think I'm doing strenuous cardio and weight training five days a week for hours at a time, but I'm certainly not. This guide is my personal take on weight loss and wellness. Commit to this process, and watch your mindset and body change!

Decide

Take a few minutes to think about what you really want to achieve for your body and why. When you get an answer that resonates with you, write it down. Then write your "I am" statement. Feel free to write as many "I am" affirmations as you like. Post them on your bathroom mirror, at your desk, on your fridge, and anywhere else that will keep you self-motivated.

The first step to obtaining your best physical body is to mentally *decide* that you not only truly want it and *deserve* it but also are committed to making it happen. Saying "We'll see what happens" or "I'll give it a try" is *not* going to cut it. You must make an absolute decision that you are going to make it happen. Once you make a firm decision, your subconscious and the universe will conspire to make it happen.

Once you set your goal, whether it's to reach a specific weight or clothing size, or to get off certain medications, write it down and post it somewhere you will see it daily. Each morning, look at it and say it. I would look at mine and say out loud "I am 130 pounds" even though I was far from it at the time. Before you reach any goal, you have to know exactly what it is. You also need to go within and determine for yourself *why* you want it.

For me, I wanted to feel lighter, look better in (and out of) my clothes, and be healthy so I could keep up with my son. I had him at forty and enjoyed my pregnancy way too much, using it as an excuse to eat anything and everything I wanted. I gained fifty pounds! But I can proudly say that I am now maintaining a weight five pounds less than my prepregnancy weight. I got the weight off and then some with the techniques I am now sharing with you.

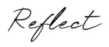

Reflect

What do you want to achieve?

_____

_____

_____

_____

_____

What is your "why"?

_____

_____

_____

_____

_____

"I Am" Statements

I am

_____

I am

_____

I am

_____

I am

_____

I am

_____

I am

_____

I am

_____

Believe

After you have made a decision to achieve a healthier body, you must now *believe* you can do it. This is how you begin to reprogram your subconscious mind. Before you go to bed, when you first wake up, and anytime you think about it during the day, visualize yourself at your goal. Now imagine how you will *feel* once you've met your goal. Sit in those feelings for a good thirty seconds at a time. Feel those feelings of accomplishment as if you're already there. It is important to see yourself reaching your goal. It must first happen in your mind.

In order to be successful, you must begin to reconnect with yourself, accept yourself fully in this present moment, and cut out *all* negative self-talk. Don't even make negative jokes about yourself because your subconscious hears everything you say and does not have a sense of humor. If you say "I'm so fat," your body will say "OK, let's stay fat," and it follows suit. If you say "I'm going to lose weight," you will perpetually be in a state of "going to." You must speak in the affirmative and in the now to invoke change. "I am achieving my best body." Changing your beliefs for the better and how you talk to yourself will begin to reprogram your subconscious. This will subsequently begin to change your habits. Also take a moment to be grateful for your body in this present moment for what it *can* do and what it has done thus far.

To reconnect to yourself and establish acceptance and trust, I highly recommend doing some mirror work. Set the timer on your phone for three to five minutes and stand about six inches from a mirror. Pick either one of your eyes to stare into in the mirror. In other words, use both of your physical eyes to stare at one eye in the mirror. Do not break eye contact. It is likely that you've probably never done this before for this amount of time. Emotions will probably start coming up. Allow them to come up. At the end of the duration, say out loud "[Your name], I see you. I accept you fully and completely. I love you." Repeat this exercise when you feel out of sorts, off balance, or disconnected from yourself.

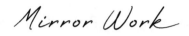

Mirror Work

What feelings came up during the three to five minutes?

_____

_____

_____

_____

_____

_____

How did you feel afterward?

_____

_____

_____

_____

_____

_____

Drink

Now that we have prepped your mind, it's time to start taking action, and I don't mean working out. The first physical thing you need to get right is your water intake. Yes, water, water, water! Our bodies are made up of at least 70 percent water. It is crucial that you are properly hydrated every day. If not, it will be extremely difficult (or impossible) to lose weight and achieve optimum health.

The key is to drink at least half of your current body weight in ounces of water per day. For example, if you are 180 pounds, you should be drinking at least ninety ounces of water per day, and more on days you exercise to replace water loss through sweat. And when I say water, I mean straight-up H_2O, not juice or soda—*water*.

Personally, I don't waste calories on beverages except for the creamer in my coffee or the occasional cocktail. How and when you drink your water is just as important as the amount. Here's the breakdown.

Drink sixteen to twenty ounces of room-temperature water within fifteen minutes of waking up in the morning. A great practice is to keep a bottle of water at your bedside, so it's right there for you to drink upon waking. Drinking this water first thing wakes up your digestive system and gets things moving, literally. For my fellow coffee drinkers, please never ever, ever let coffee be the first thing in your stomach in the morning. By doing that, you are destroying your stomach lining. Everyone needs to start with water—again, within fifteen minutes of waking up.

As a bonus, add a little lemon or lime juice to your water.

Drink your water separately from your meals. If you are cooking the meal, drink during your prep time. Aim to drink sixteen to twenty ounces at least twenty to thirty minutes *before* mealtimes. Now, of course you can have a few sips with your meal to help wash it down, but the bulk of the water should be consumed twenty to thirty minutes before eating. If you are drinking while eating, drink warm water instead of cold water, as cold fluids will begin to solidify fat and oils from the food you're eating. When you eat and simultaneously have a *large* glass of water or what have you, it interferes with digestion and the proper assimilation of nutrients from the food.

Here's another reason why water is so important. Did you know that your intestines can hold anywhere from five to twenty pounds of feces? A lot of that can be alleviated by drinking enough water. When your body is dehydrated, the intestines will, in essence, absorb the moisture from the food you eat. This, then, makes it more difficult for food to travel through the intestines, and that waste becomes compacted in your system. So yes, some people are literally full of sh*t! This excess waste in your system causes a buildup of toxicity, which begins to have a negative effect on the body and immune system.

At a minimum, you should be pooping at least once a day, *every* day. When you start eating fewer processed foods and drinking more water, you'll likely go two to three times per day. This is normal and optimum.

So now that you know how much to drink and when to drink it, let's up the ante. Water holds vibration (frequency or sound). I speak affirmations into my water. For example, I might say "I am healthy, whole, and complete," "I am in the best shape of my life," "I am abundant," or "I am a magnet for blessings." At a minimum, I say "thank you" and "I love you" into it. Speak life into your water before you drink it. Remember that your body is at least 70 percent water, so please be mindful of what you speak and think about yourself. *Your body is listening and will do what you command and believe to be true.*

Determine Your
Daily Water Goal

Current weight _____ divided by 2
= _____ ounces of water daily.

I am committed to drinking _____
ounces of water per day.

Eat/Fast

Regardless of the food lifestyle you sub-scribe to—whether vegan, pescatarian, vegetarian, or "I eat everything"—it is important to give your digestive system proper rest. At a minimum, I recommend fasting for at least twelve hours per day. By fasting, I mean no snacking or eating during a prolonged window of time. Water and unsweetened tea are OK during your fasting window. Personally, I aim to not have anything except water from 8:00 p.m. to 8:00 a.m. based on my schedule. For those who work nights, your fasting window will be during the day, including a few hours before and after your sleep period. I also make sure my last meal or snack is at least three to four hours before bedtime. This twelve-hour fasting window works well while in the maintenance phase.

If you are in a weight-loss phase, I recommend increasing your fasting window to fourteen to sixteen hours. This is called intermittent fasting. For example, when I'm trying to drop a few pounds, I'll only eat between noon to 8:00 p.m. I do still have coffee in the morning at least thirty minutes after my water, of course. Some may argue that having coffee with creamer and/or sweetener isn't true intermittent fasting, but, hey, this works for me. So it would likely work for you. (My coffee drinkers can jump for joy.)

The longer fasting window will force your body to burn more stored fat for energy because there is no food coming in to burn. Regardless of your food lifestyle, aim to eat whole foods with ingredients you can pronounce.

Avoid or at least limit processed foods as much as possible, and be mindful of your sugar intake.

Before eating, I bless my food by saying "Thank you for keeping me in perfect health, in perfect shape, and at the perfect weight." Why? Because water holds vibration, and there is some amount of water in your food. You also want to be mindful while eating. *Slow down.* Savor every bite by chewing slowly until it's basically liquid in your mouth. Too many of us rush through meals and barely chew before we swallow, which strains the digestive system. Sometimes we eat so fast that we immediately want more—not because we're still hungry, but because we want to continue enjoying the deliciousness. Slow down.

Determine Your
Fasting Window

Example:

I am generally awake from 6:45 a.m. to 11:00 p.m.

My fasting window is 8:00 p.m. to 8:00 a.m.

When I'm intending to lose weight, my fasting window is 8:00 p.m. to 12:00 noon the next day.

Your fasting window:

I am generally awake from _____ a.m./p.m.

to _____ a.m./p.m.

My fasting window will be _____ a.m./p.m.

to _____ a.m./p.m.

Rest

In order to keep your body and mind functioning well, you also need adequate rest. I feel my best when I've had seven to eight hours of sleep. However, some people function well with only five to six hours of sleep. I am not one of those people. Determine what feels good for you, and aim to gift yourself with that amount of rest on most nights. Try to go to bed around the same time every night to get your body into a rhythm.

If you have trouble falling asleep, try turning off electronics thirty minutes before bed. Do some reading, deep-breathing exercises, or a guided meditation for sleep. Create a ritual for yourself so your mind and body know it's time to settle down for a good night's rest.

When you are drifting off to sleep is a great time to reprogram your subconscious. You can do this by reciting your "I am" affirmations silently to yourself, listening to healing frequencies, or using guided hypnosis from a trusted source. Healing frequencies are particular frequencies of sound that are used to stimulate the brain to promote healing in the body and mind. This may also be referred to as sound therapy. Guided hypnosis or hypnotherapy is a form of psychotherapy in which a person is guided by an expert into a deep state of relaxation and then given statements to help reprogram the person's subconscious. You can find healing frequencies and guided hypnosis sessions on YouTube or on various meditation apps; two of my favorite apps are Aura and Insight Timer. As a bonus, you can also create a recording using your phone of your own voice speaking your affirmations and intentions. Then listen to this nightly as you fall asleep.

Reflect

**I feel my best when I have at least
_____ hours of sleep.**

**I am committed to gifting myself with at
least _____ hours of sleep per night.**

Exercise

Last but not least, exercise! Actually, it kind of *is* least because everything else we've already covered is about 80 percent of weight loss and maintenance. Exercise is that last 20 percent. Aim to move your body for at least thirty minutes a day. A few days of the week, your exercise should be more intense, where you're getting your heart rate up and you're sweating. On other days, do something gentler like going for a walk or simply putting on your favorite music and dancing. Moving your body and celebrating what it can do should be a fun and joyful experience. Find a few things you *enjoy* so that it is easier to be *consistent*. Then figure out how to use those activities to increase your cardio endurance, strength, and flexibility. Consistency is key!

Regardless of the exercises you do, here's my secret to a strong, sexy core. Throughout the day, whenever I think about it, I contract my abdominal muscles. I do this when I'm brushing my teeth, washing dishes, going for a walk, waiting in line at the grocery store, and most certainly while exercising. I engage my abs continually, which helps to passively build that muscle without a ton of actual ab exercises. So whenever you think about it, squeeze your abs while continuing to breathe!

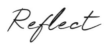

Reflect

Types of exercise I enjoy (or think I would):

_____

_____

_____

_____

_____

Types of exercise I think my body needs:

_____

_____

_____

_____

_____

I am committed to moving my body _____ minutes a day, _____ days a week.

Conclusion

I hope that I have opened your mind to new concepts to help you on your journey to your best self. This guide is a culmination of what I have learned about health and wellness in the past twenty-plus years, condensed into its simplest form.

First, you must change your mindset about what your body is capable of and believe you can achieve your best self. Decide to commit to the process. Love yourself by only speaking positively about your body. Remember, our bodies are mostly water, so love yourself enough to drink all the water your body needs. Fast for at least twelve hours every twenty-four-hour cycle to give your digestive system a break and burn stored fat. Eat whole, unprocessed foods. The body heals during rest, so get plenty of sleep! Move your body daily: go for long walks in nature, dance in front of a mirror, take time to stretch, find a group fitness class you enjoy, or go to the gym!

Remember that this is a process and that change takes time. Believe in yourself. Show yourself grace if you fall off, but do be accountable to yourself to get right back on track. Better yet, find a friend or two to embark on this journey with, and hold each other accountable.

You deserve to feel good, inside and out! Believe in yourself! You can do it!

About the Author

Erika Washington (formerly Erika Gary) was born and raised in Piscataway, New Jersey. She received her BS in electrical engineering from Howard University, and her MS in electrical engineering from North Carolina A&T State University. Erika is currently a divorced mom of one son, and she resides in Maryland. Since childhood, she has had a passion for dance, exercise, and self-improvement. She has received fitness certifications through AFAA (Athletics and Fitness Association of America) and was certified by the legendary Billy Blanks as a Tae Bo® instructor.